The Habit System

10 Powerful Habits *For*

Sustainable Leanness

KEITH HILDEBRAND

CONTENTS

THE HABIT SYSTEM

INTRODUCTION

First and foremost, thank you for purchasing the Habit System book.

This book was created in order to help:

- Those who have tried to diet in the past and have experienced failure

- Those with little to no experience with fat loss who are looking to get started

- Those who need to revamp/improve their overall eating habits

What you will find inside is a system of 10 skills that will help you improve your eating habits and finally reach your fat loss goals. Whether you are an absolute beginner or have some level of experience with dieting, this system will teach you what is most important for losing fat and keeping it off in the long term. The system is not a fad diet that is meant to provide a short term fix. Instead, it focuses on practicing key habits that can be used for the rest of your life to successfully manage your weight.

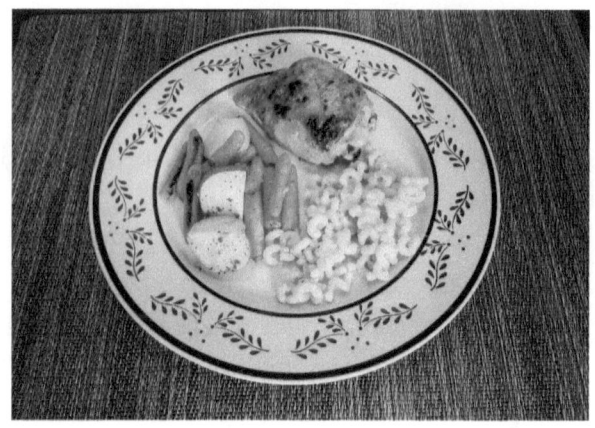

WHY THIS SYSTEM IS DIFFERENT

Losing weight is tough and keeping that weight off in the long term is even tougher. Despite the fact that there is an entire industry built around helping people lose weight, most fail to ever reach their fat loss goals and it is easy to see why. In our opinion, one key issue is that most diets are just too difficult to stick to especially for long periods of time. Many popular diets require complete avoidance of certain food groups and offer little flexibility making adherence difficult. More importantly, most diets do not provide a progressive system that actually teaches you skills that you can continue using in the future. That is why we created the Habit System.

With the Habit System below you will practice implementing one habit at a time until you have successfully mastered it. After that you will begin working on additional habits until you become proficient with the entire system. This creates more of a sustainable lifestyle change for users versus promoting "crash" behaviors, such as cutting out all carbohydrates from your diet or exercising seven days per week. Please understand that the key to making this system successful is **practice** and **consistency**. Weight loss and weight management are skills that need to be learned and developed. You would not expect to be able to speak a new language fluently without learning it and practicing. You also would not expect to be able to hit a three point shot the first time you pick up a basketball. Weight loss is no different and understanding this will save you a lot of time and frustration.

HOW TO USE THIS BOOK

In order to get the most benefit from this system, we highly recommend reading through the entire document first to better understand exactly what habits you will be working on. Once you have read through the habits and feel that you understand them, it is time to begin practicing.

Each habit should be practiced individually unless you feel that you are able to handle more than one at a time. In the "Worksheets" section of this book, you will find a 10 day Habit Log worksheet for your use that you can make multiple copies of. Select your first habit and begin practicing this habit daily. Use the Habit Log to track your daily progress/adherence by placing a check mark (√) in the box of the habit(s) you practice each day (also write the date at the top). As you begin to work on additional habits be sure to continue checking off the previous habits each day as you should continue to implement them as well. A space for "notes" is also provided below every habit listed. Use this space to log any additional information about the habits for your future reference (ex: difficulty with a particular habit, unforeseen issues, explanations, partial adherence, etc.).

We recommend practicing each habit for a period of 10 - 20 days. It is perfectly fine if you need to work on certain habits for longer than

20 days as some are more difficult than others. Please keep in mind that these habits need to be viewed as skills that require practice. Practice implementing each habit for as long as necessary in order for you to feel that you have mastered them and can follow them consistently.

In terms of order to follow, we highly suggest beginning with Habits 1, 2 and 3. These three habits will be the high impact fundamental habits that will lay the foundation for your fat loss success. Once you have successfully implemented the first three, you can choose which habits to work on next based on your individual needs and preferences. There is not a specific order that will be beneficial for everyone to follow as each person's needs will vary. Without assessing your dieting history, current habits and preferences we cannot recommend a universal order to follow. By utilizing the Food Journal as presented in Habit 1 however, you will begin to recognize the glaring issues that exist with your eating habits. Take advantage of the steps presented in Habit 1 to help uncover the areas that truly require your focus.

A few important points before you begin

In order to help you successfully implement the habit system, we would like to discuss a few important points before you begin.

MEALS AND SNACKS

As a general rule of thumb we recommend that you consume three to four meals and one to two snacks each day while following the habit system. We find that this is typically ideal for most people and does not create any large periods of time where overwhelming hunger can sneak up on you and derail your progress. Habits 4, 5, 6 and 10 will show you how to create meals that will keep you feeling full while helping you to reduce your total calorie intake. Habit 3 will explain how to improve the way you eat your meals so that you eat just enough and avoid consuming excess calories. If you need to eat more or less than the recommended amount of meals and snacks due to personal preferences or schedule limitations that is perfectly alright. Just be sure to stick to the habit guidelines to ensure that you are taking the proper actions to help you reach your fat loss goals.

WHOLE FOODS

As part of your efforts to improve your collective eating habits, including more whole foods and less processed foods in your diet is going to be important. The habits listed in the system below will help you do so on their own however, you need to be actively aware of the quality of your foods. Overly processed foods that are made from refined ingredients and artificial substances can hinder your fat loss efforts and neg-

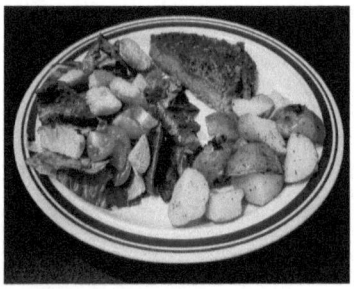

atively affect your health. Processed foods typically contain added sugar and refined "simple" carbohydrates which add extra calories to your meals and spike blood sugar and insulin levels. They are also engineered to be hyper rewarding to the brain (with added sugar, salt and fat) which can easily lead to over-consumption. Processed foods are usually extremely low in essential nutrients and fiber compared to whole foods as well as they are stripped away during processing.

Whole foods are ideal as they are typically nutrient dense and generally contain less calories than processed foods. They also require more energy to eat and digest with one study showing that whole foods burned twice as many calories as processed foods. Do your best to choose foods that are closest to their natural state with minimal added ingredients. Choose baked potatoes over instant mashed potatoes, Greek yogurt over sweetened yogurts/parfaits, fresh meats and fish over deli meats and fish sticks. Focusing on the perimeter of the grocery store (produce, meats, dairy, etc.) when shopping is extremely helpful to ensure that the bulk of your groceries are whole foods as well.

EXERCISE CONSIDERATIONS

While the primary driver of weight loss is a sustained caloric deficit (eating less calories than you are burning), exercise can be an incredibly useful tool to help speed up your progress. It is definitely not required as you will likely experience noticeable weight loss from the Habit System alone however exercise will work synergistically with the system to improve your chances of success. Our general recommendation is to exercise three to four days per week with roughly 65%-75% of that effort being focused on progressive strength training. The remaining training time can be used for long distance cardio, high intensity interval training (HIIT), classes or any exercise style of your choice. Please keep in mind that these are our general recommendations for what will likely work *best* and that any exercise style that you can consistently complete will help to improve your results. Pick what you enjoy and practice it consistently!

While everyone's individual needs and abilities are different, we believe progressive strength training will help your fat loss efforts tremendously. Strength training is important because it allows you to burn a substantial amount of calories, increase muscle mass (that will burn additional calories) and slowly shape your body to your liking. As we cannot make specific exercise recommendations without assessing each individual, only perform exercises that you are comfortable with that can be completed with safe and proper form. Similar to the habits presented in the system below, **practice** and **consistency** are going to be key for success with this as well. If you are not currently exercising regularly, work to slowly add multiple workout days to your weekly schedule at your own pace.

LET'S TALK ABOUT YOUR CURRENT DIET

Addressing your diet is *extremely* important when it comes to seeing tangible changes in your physique, performance and/or health. You can work as hard as you want to in the gym, however you are not going to see optimal results unless you understand and adjust what foods you are putting into your body. In addition to adjusting the types of foods you are eating, you are likely going to have to change the way you look at "dieting" altogether.

WHY YOUR DIET IS NOT WORKING

If you chose to read this book, it is probably safe to say that whatever diet you are currently following or have followed in the past is not working and that is totally fine! If losing fat and getting in better shape were that simple, everyone would look amazing and personal trainers would be out of business. Unfortunately, that is not the case and most people struggle to shed excess body fat in the long term. Before we begin implementing steps that will work though, we think it is going to be extremely helpful for you to understand why your dieting efforts have not been giving you the results that you want.

To put the general public's struggles with dieting into context, Dr. Layne Norton (PhD in Nutritional Sciences) offers three statistics that will show you that you are not alhone:

- Research data shows that of the people that lose weight, 80% will have gained that weight back within a year.

- Of that 80% who gained their weight back, nearly half will have put on more weight than they initially lost.

- On average, the number of times that you try to diet in your life is directly proportional to the amount of fat you gain during your life time.

Statistics like these make it clear that many people are failing when it comes to their diet. One might even come to the conclusion that dieting ultimately makes you fatter. Dieting **does not** make you fatter, but <u>the way that most people diet</u> sets them up for failure and tremendous rebound/subsequent fat gain. Why does this happen? Let's discuss the multiple factors involved.

SHORT-TERM FOCUS

One major issue with the way most people diet is their expectation of how much fat they should be losing in a set (usually short) period of time. In today's world especially, people demand instant gratification and expect results overnight. People's expectations are typically no different when it comes to losing body fat and keeping it off. We're going to break the bad news to you right now before we go any further: it does not work that way.

Can you lose a large amount of bodyweight in a relatively short amount of time? Absolutely. You can crash diet and see the numbers on your scale drop rather quickly. You might want to consider what that entails though first.

- *Severe restrictions.* If you want to see drastic results then you are going to need to make drastic changes over night. There is no time to develop a comprehensive system of long lasting healthy habits because that cannot be accomplished over the span of only four to six weeks. You will need to cut out many of the foods/drinks you love immediately which can cause overwhelming cravings and could potentially develop and/or reinforce disordered eating patterns. Do you see yourself being able to do that six months or one year from now? How about five years?

- *Substantially less calories.* Continuing with the necessity of severe restrictions, calories are going to have to be cut quickly and drastically. The more weight loss desired (in a short period), the more calories need to be cut because ultimately weight loss is an equation of calories in versus calories out (generally speaking, although there are many other factors that can come into play). With a limited time frame, you are not going to be able to slowly and gradually drop those calories to ensure adherence. So let's say you can maintain your current body weight (not lose weight or gain weight) by eating 2,300 calories per day. You will likely need to immediately cut your daily caloric intake down to the 1,500-1,800 range (a significant drop) which can be extremely tough to stick to.

- *Losing more than just fat.* When working towards fat loss, the goal is to lose as much fat as possible while maintaining as much muscle as possible. The more muscle you have, the stronger your metabolism will be, that is why strength training is important for fat loss efforts. When you rush weight loss, the dramatic cut in calories causes you to lose fat pretty quickly but you are also going to lose muscle mass along with it. With the loss of muscle mass comes a reduction in metabolic rate, reduction in total body strength, decreases in energy expenditure and less strong curves or dense muscle that ultimately shapes your body into the physique you desire.

IT IS NOT MAINTAINABLE

Another very important component of a diet is its maintainability. Are you able to follow that diet for more than just a few weeks or months? The reason this is so important is because the research data tells us that if the diet you are following is not maintainable and you cannot stay relatively consistent with it in the long term, you are going to fail. If you cannot see yourself following the diet you are on six months, two years or five years from now, you have to rethink what you are doing because *it will likely fail*. Why waste your time on something that you cannot see yourself using years down the line? You ultimately want to make your "diet" become your standard practice of daily eating, not a finite period of suffering that you need to fight to get through. This is why a habit based program can be much more beneficial for long term success.

Also many of the popular diets out there are too restrictive for people to follow for long periods as they demonize certain foods as "unhealthy". Obviously everyone is different and some diets work better than others for particular people.

However, any diet that tells you a certain food is off limits and restricted is likely not going to be maintainable for most people. If you really enjoy eating ice cream and your diet says that you cannot have ice cream in any amount because it's "unhealthy", how long do you think you can realistically comply? Moderation is the key (as you will see), not total restriction.

LOOKING FOR THE MAGIC PILL

Too many people are looking for that one magic supplement or product that is going to finally help them reach their goals. There are plenty of them out there too: body wraps, diet pills, creams, cleanses, etc. It is almost scary actually how many people get suckered into purchasing expensive supplements or products truly believing that this is what they have been missing out on. The sad truth is, most of the time you are completely wasting your money. Almost every single weight loss supplement out there is nearly useless and overpriced. You would save an incredible amount of money and time if you focused your efforts on improving your eating habits instead. These products also do not address the underlying issues with people's eating habits and choices. Again we hate to be the bearers of bad news, but losing weight and getting into better shape truly does boil down to putting in the work and being consistent. Do not be overwhelmed though! While that may appear to be too time intensive and challenging, as you read on you will see that it is really not as hard as you thought.

Now that we have addressed some of the major reasons why your dieting efforts have not been working, it is time to start discussing and implementing steps that do.

THE
HABIT
SYSTEM

HABIT #1: FOOD JOURNAL

Begin using a food journal for a minimum of twenty days to track everything that you eat and drink. If possible, continue to maintain your food journal until you have mastered all 10 habits. Key information to include:

- *Food/drink consumed*

- *Portion size*

- *Time it was consumed*

- *Why you ate/drank it and what you were feeling/doing at the time*

The food journal is a simple yet very important tool for those that are looking to improve their eating habits. Your food journal provides you with the raw data that you need to plan a successful strategy, track your progress and make adjustments along the way. The journal is **not** a moral compass, it is not there to tell you whether your meals are good or bad, healthy or unhealthy. Instead it serves as clear direct feedback about whether you are taking actions that bring you closer to your goal or further from it, and that is it.

THE HABIT SYSTEM

The primary benefits you will get from using a food journal, even if it is only for the 20 day period are:

- To identify your exact starting point. You likely know how much you weigh currently however you probably do not keep track of your eating habits with much detail. This will serve to paint an accurate picture of how you are currently eating and will help you identify key areas where you are making mistakes.

- To determine what factors are coming into play when you make your food choices. Did you simply just feel like eating that McDonald's meal or was it the only quick option available at the time? Take a second to analyze the thought process behind your meal choices. We can improve bad habits, however you must first identify them.

- For reference in the future to see just how much your diet and habits have changed.

You do not need to list the amount of calories

and macronutrients (carbs, fat and protein) that each food/drink contains if you do not have the time however you should list everything consumed, even the amount of water you are drinking. Be sure to also include any notes that you can about why you chose the particular meal/snack. Was this meal planned in advance or was it chosen due to time constraints and/or location? Did you eat an entire bag of chips? Why? Was it because you were upset/stressed or came home from work absolutely starving? Identifying the reasons behind your food choices will help tremendously and will show you what areas you need to improve.

A detailed food journal example is shown below (blank template in the "Worksheets" section):

Meal (Include time)	Food/Beverage (Type and amount)	Calories	Protein (Grams)	Carbs (Grams)	Fat (Grams)	Notes
Breakfast 6:00 AM	4 Whole Eggs	280	24	0	20	Scrambled with pepper
	1/2 Cup Oatmeal	150	5	27	3	With cinnamon
	1 Cup Black Coffee	0	0	0	0	No sugar/cream
	Meal Notes: Woke up starving, felt full after meal for hours. Ate slowly, controlled portions easily.					
Snack 10:00 AM	1 Ounce Habanero BBQ Almonds	170	6	5	15	
	Meal Notes: Struggled to make it to 10 AM for snack. Held me over sufficiently until lunch. Somewhat filling.					
Lunch 12:00 PM	1 Panera Chicken Caesar Salad	430	28	15	27	Used about 80% of dressing
	1 Cup Diet Coke	0	0	0	0	Switched to diet instead of full sugar
	Meal Notes: Was in a rush and had to grab a quick meal. Best "healthy" option I could find. Felt full and satiated after.					
Snack 2:00 PM	2 Jalapeno Cheddar Cheese Sticks	180	10	0	14	
	Meal Notes: Planned snack, and they're filling. Easily can make it until dinner time after eating.					
Dinner 5:00 PM	9 Ounce Porkchop	180	39	15	6	Lightly seasoned
	1 Cup Sweet Potatoes	159	2	37	0	With cinnamon and light butter
	1 Cup Green Beans	44	2	10	0	Plain
	2 Cups Diet Iced Tea	0	0	0	0	
	Meal Notes: Planned dinner, cooked in 30 minutes. Ate slowly until I felt full. No cravings for dessert tonight.					

Note: Tracking calories and macronutrients (protein, carbs and fat) is optional.

THE HABIT SYSTEM

Once you have completed 20 days of logging your food and beverages, it is time to inspect your eating habits. After you review what you have consumed, sit down and ask yourself the following questions (and be honest):

- *Where did I make mistakes*? Are you including protein and vegetables into any of your meals? Are you consuming foods/drinks with incredibly high amounts of calories? You don't need to get overly detailed; instead just try to identify the major glaring issues.

- *When did I consume "unhealthy" meals/snacks/beverages*? (Unhealthy, for our purposes, will mean foods high in calories, high in sugar, low in nutrients, and/or overly processed). Is there a common time each day that you are doing this?

- *What truly led me to consume these "unhealthy" items*? Was it because you simply craved it or was that your only option at the time? Were you running on little sleep? Were you upset? The reasons matter and will help you figure out what habits are truly hindering your progress.

At the very least, aim to keep a detailed food journal for at least a 20 day period. If you find that you are able to with no issues, we highly recommend continuing this habit until you have mastered all 10 habits. Don't worry, you will not need to journal your food for the rest of your life. However, we believe that practicing this habit for an extended period of time can be extremely beneficial to clients. It will help you pinpoint exactly what mistakes you are making, help you understand why you are making them and allow you to keep a detailed history of your progress for reference in the future. Maintaining a consistent food journal will also be incredibly helpful to successfully execute the other nine habits. Finally, it allows you to learn about the foods you eat (ingredients, nutritional information, portions, etc.) and how your body responds to them (body weight, hunger, energy levels, etc.). The more information you can learn and keep for reference the better!

HABIT #2: PREPARE! PICK A SET DAY TO PLAN/SHOP/ COOK

Pick one day each week to plan out your meals/snacks for the week, shop for all necessary ingredients and to cook/prepare/portion any meals/ snacks that you can. Weekends may work best.

If you are going to take your fat loss efforts seriously, you have to do your best to be as prepared as you can ahead of time. Preparation and strategy are **incredibly** important, especially when it comes to fat loss, because they help prevent you from putting yourself in situations where you will need to rely solely on will power. Relying on will power alone is a recipe for disaster and we want to avoid that as much as possible. Mistakes are also very easy to make without a plan to follow, especially considering the unpredictability of most people's days.

To illustrate this point, imagine that you wake up on a Monday morning and decide to skip breakfast because you want to lose weight. Your current understanding of dieting lead you to the decision to skip consuming these calories because in your mind, less calories = less body fat. Then you get to work and your hunger starts to really kick in. You do not have any go-to healthy snack so instead you head down to the office vending machine and demolish a bag of chips and a sugary beverage (soda, Gatorade, juice, sweetened iced tea, etc.). This snack holds you over until roughly noon when you decide to go eat lunch. Since you did not prepare a lunch ahead of time and you are crunched for time (everyone is busy and not everyone has the time to take a full lunch break), you run to the closest fast food establishment you can find. Now you are not even halfway through your day and you likely have consumed a substantial amount of processed foods rich in carbohydrates and fat with little protein/fiber/micronutrients.

A week after that, you decide to prepare ahead

of time and begin your week with a solid strategy. You shopped for food on Sunday so you had eggs, peppers, onions, spinach and oatmeal portioned and ready to be prepared for breakfast on Monday morning (veggie filled scrambled eggs with a small bowl of oatmeal covered in cinnamon is a delicious breakfast option). You feel full, energized and able to focus on your work until about 10 AM when you reach for two handfuls of almonds (our personal favorite: Blue Diamond almonds). These almonds keep you full and satiated until lunch time when you eat the leftovers of your lean dinner from the night before. Because you planned ahead and implemented a well thought out strategy, your chances of failing decreased dramatically and you were able to stick to your plan. This is why preparation is critical for your success.

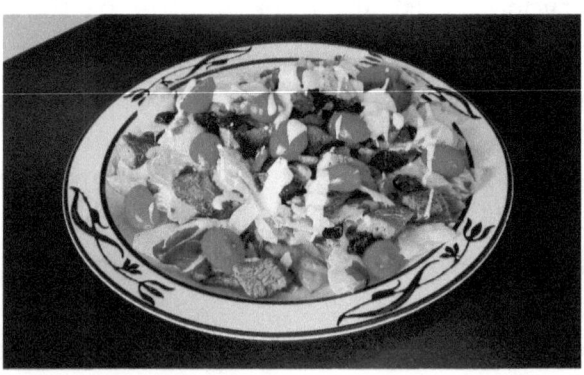

How to Prepare

Designate a specific day of the week as your weekly "Preparation Day". This will be the most important day of your week where you will focus on engineering the next seven days to ensure fat loss success. On this day your "workout" is preparation and planning, and that is it. Your sole focus will be planning meals/snacks, shopping for ingredients and cooking/preparing/portioning any foods that you can ahead of time for the coming week.

Your first step is to sit down and take the time to think through all of the meals/snacks you are going to eat over the next seven days. Do your best to plan out as many of these meals as you can and identify which ingredients you will need in order to prepare them. Please understand that in the beginning this may seem challenging to implement (and that's totally alright). You are not expected to be able to successfully plan every single meal from the start; it is going to take time to get to that point. Instead of overwhelming yourself and trying to tackle all of your meals at once, just practice getting *one meal right at a time* at your own pace for as long as necessary. Pick one meal (ex: Monday Dinner) and practice these three steps to help you master it:

1. *Plan the meal*: Decide what you are going to eat (use the Habit System as your guide to craft meals), when you are going to eat it, what ingredients you need in order to prepare it and how you will prepare it.

2. *Execute*: Purchase the ingredients and cook/prepare/portion any that you can ahead of time. Meats can be cooked in bulk, vegetables can be chopped/organized and snacks can be portioned/packaged. When meal time arrives, finish any last preparations and enjoy the meal you've put together. Be sure to log this meal in your food journal with all necessary information.

3. *Review your journal*: Review the information you logged in your food journal. Inspect portion sizes, calories and meal notes. Think about how much food you needed to eat to get to the point of feeling comfortable and satisfied

(not stuffed). Think about how long the particular meal kept you feeling full for and if it needs to be modified to extend that period. Did you follow the Fit Path Habits with this meal?

Once you have practiced a particular meal consistently and feel comfortable with the preparation/execution of it, begin working on an additional meal. The idea will be to slowly keep building your planning/preparation skills until you reach the point where you can map out your entire week with ease. All you need to do is start with just one meal. It does not matter which meal you start with either. If you struggle with eating a healthy breakfast that keeps you full for hours, start there! If your food journal has shown you that you make the biggest mistakes with your dinner meals, work on getting those right first! Eventually you will reach the point where you are able to easily plan out the majority of your meals for the week and prepare for them appropriately. It is just going to take practice.

Please also note that by planning ahead, you can virtually avoid any issues that may potentially pop up and knock you off course. Here are a few major obstacles that people deal with during the week that can sometimes instantly derail their progress (but will no longer derail yours):

- Picking up groceries after work to prepare for dinner - If you list, purchase and organize all of your ingredients on Sunday/Monday this problem is easily avoided. You will also avoid the possibility that your time to purchase groceries during the week is cut short due to staying late at work and/or running into unforeseen traffic.

- Significant other who does not want to eat your "healthier" meals - You can work together to create lean meals that they will enjoy as well or you can figure out how to eat separate meals and make it work for the both of you. Either way, you have addressed it ahead of time and avoided potential failure.

- Eating out frequently at work - Now you can inspect menus ahead of time and select healthier choices instead of winging it when you get there. Many popular restaurants now include nutritional information on their menus as well to help you decide what's best.

Tips to increase adherence:

- *Prepare shopping lists ahead of time organized by either food type or by meal.* While this suggestion may seem overly-obvious, you would be surprised by how many people simply show up to the grocery store with zero preparation at all. Don't set yourself up for failure!

- *Start small.* As with all of these habits, they truly take practice and patience. If you are not comfortable or able to plan out all of your meals and snacks for the week at once, that's no problem! Work on what you can handle for now and slowly try to build upon that each week. If you are looking for a reasonable first step to begin working on, we suggest focusing on your grocery list. This will get you in the habit of thinking ahead and isn't too overwhelming for most people.

- *Whenever possible, cook/prepare meats and vegetables in bulk ahead of time.* If you know you will be using a particular meat multiple times throughout the week (chicken for salad and stir fry, lean ground turkey for tacos and chili) then season and cook all of it at one time. If you know you'll be adding a variety of veggies to your breakfast eggs, chop and portion them all so there is zero preparation required in the morning. The more you can prepare in advance the better.

HABIT #3: EAT SLOWLY AND STOP ONCE YOU REACH YOUR "SATISFACTION ZONE"

Practice and implement the following strategies to improve the way you are eating your meals and to help develop better mindful eating habits:

- *Eat until you feel satisfied/comfortable instead of stuffed/uncomfortable.*

- *Eat your protein source and vegetables first before your carbohydrates and fats.*

- *After each bite you take during your meals, take a drink (preferably of water or a low-calorie beverage) and wait 15 seconds before your next bite.*

- *Place your utensils down after each bite and do not pick them back up until your food is chewed thoroughly and swallowed.*

- *Work towards hitting a total meal time of 15-20 minutes with each meal (eat slowly).*

- *Commit to eating free of distractions (turn off your TV and stay off of your cell phone).*

Mindful eating habits, such as those listed above, can be incredibly helpful for weight loss. While some may initially seem overwhelming, these simple steps can deliver powerful results on their own *if you practice them*. The primary goal is to adjust the way you are eating your meals so that you are consuming them more slowly and better recognizing when you are actually satisfied (instead of overly full). Most people eat their meals far too quickly and completely miss their body's signals of satisfaction. These steps will help you avoid this mistake and give you a better understanding of just how much you need to eat to successfully manage your hunger.

Habit #3: Eat Slowly and Stop Once You Reach Your "Satisfaction Zone"

By simply eating your meals more slowly, you can improve your digestion, lose/maintain weight easier and gain better control over your hunger. One of the most important reasons you will want to eat your meals more slowly is that it gives your body enough time to recognize that you are full. We are all guilty of eating our meals too quickly, it is easy to do especially when your time is limited. Your body requires roughly 15 - 20 minutes though to send the signals of satiety (satisfaction) indicating that you have eaten enough. By simply slowing down the pace with which you eat your food (using the steps above), you can easily prevent yourself from overeating and consuming excess calories. When you eat too quickly, it is incredibly easy to over shoot your calorie needs because you have not allowed your body enough time to let you know that it is full/satisfied. The bottom line: work on extending your meal times!

In addition to eating more slowly you should focus on eating **just enough** food to satisfy your hunger and feel comfortable. That is the point where you want to stop eating, once you reach what we call the "satisfaction zone". When you reach the satisfaction zone with a meal you should feel comfortable, energized and be able to go for a walk without having to wait for your food to digest. You should not feel bloated, uncomfortable, overly full and deprived of energy. Your stomach should not hurt and you should not feel tired. Hunger should also remain non-existent for a few hours after you eat (if it does not you likely fell just short of reaching your satisfaction zone). It will take time but once you recognize just how much food you require to reach satisfaction, it will become much easier to identify when you are eating too little or too much.

Listen to your body's feedback to help you identify where exactly your satisfaction zone lies. It may take you time to figure out just where that zone is for you but it is going to be important to identify. That zone may begin at eight bites of a particular meal for you while it begins with six bites for someone else. It may end at 12 bites for you and 11 bites for another person. Regardless, you will slowly begin to recognize your sweet spot of satisfaction that will allow you to create a calorie deficit (burning more calories than you are consuming) while successfully managing your hunger. Eating free of distractions will also help you better recognize when you reach the satisfaction zone. Watching TV and scrolling through Facebook on your phone while you eat diverts your attention away from the meal and your hunger/satisfaction awareness. Your focus should be on your meal, how it tastes and how you feel after each bite, so do your best to re-move any distractions that shift your attention!

We suggest practicing only one or two of the strategies listed above at a time unless you feel confident that you can handle more. You will likely experience the most success beginning with either "taking a drink after each bite and waiting 15 seconds" or "placing your utensils down after each bite". They are incredibly sim-ple and easy to follow and will help you slowly work your way up to a total meal time of ap-proximately 20 minutes. Once you feel that you have mastered these two strategies, begin working on another. Before you know it, you will be able to completely change the way you con-sume your meals for the better!

Tips to increase adherence:
- *Set a timer* (you can use your phone for this) for 15-20 minutes each time you sit

down to eat a meal. Do your best not to finish eating until the full time is up. Monitoring the countdown of the timer while you eat will also help you set an appropriate eating pace.

- *Be mindful of how much you chew.* The more you can chew your food the better, so do your best to ensure that all food is thoroughly broken down before you swallow it. Also aim to include fibrous foods in your meals that require significant chewing (vegetables, fruits, nuts, etc.).

- *Avoid extreme hunger.* When you are hit with ravenous hunger, it can be incredibly tough to eat your meals slowly. Try to keep healthy low calorie snacks close by so that you can avoid intense overwhelming urges to binge eat and consume excess calories.

HABIT #4: EAT MORE VEGETABLES

Increase your daily consumption of vegetables to at least six cups per day.

Regardless of your goals, consuming plenty of vegetables is important for your health (high vegetable intake has been shown to reduce the risk of cancer, cardiovascular disease, coronary heart disease, stroke, diabetes and obesity). Vegetables are filled with a plethora of vitamins, minerals and fiber, but most importantly (for fat loss efforts) the majority of vegetables contain a very minimal amount of calories compared to most foods. You will fill up much quicker and fight off hunger much longer by eating 400 calories from vegetables as opposed to 400 calories from chocolate cake. That is why they are perfect for helping individuals lose weight as vegetables allow you to add volume to your meals to make them more filling and satisfying without a high calorie total.

Adding multiple cups of veggies to your diet alone can have an incredibly positive impact on your weight. By simply eating more vegetables, you can reduce your daily calorie intake almost effortlessly. They will help you reach fullness more quickly and fight off hunger for longer periods after meals. They are tasty and satisfying, providing an easy tool that can be used to prevent excess calorie consumption with each meal. They are also an excellent and delicious snack choice.

The chart below shows many popular vegetables and their respective amount of calories per cup. Use this chart if you choose to track calories or would like a rough estimate of the calorie content of your vegetables.

Vegetable	Calories (per cup)	Vegetable	Calories (per cup)
Cilantro	4	Tomatoes	32
Arugula	5	Turnips	36
Spinach	7	Brussel sprouts	38
Romaine lettuce	8	Squash	39
Celery	14	Sweet red peppers	39
Mushrooms	15	Carrots	52
Cucumber	16	Leeks	54
Radishes	19	Beets	58
Eggplant	20	Chili peppers	60
Zucchini	20	Onions	67
Cabbage	21	Parsnips	100
Cauliflower	25	Sweet potatoes	114
Asparagus	27	Potatoes	116
Green peppers	30	Green peas	117
Pumpkin	30	Yellow sweet corn	132
Broccoli	31	Yam	177

Tips to increase adherence:

- *Similar to the other habits, work on implementing this slowly.* If you are currently consuming little to no vegetables, try aiming to eat 1-2 cups per day for the first few weeks. Once you can consistently do so, increase your total amount by another 1-2 cups until you hit the six cup minimum.

- *Don't just eat your vegetables as a side at lunch/dinner!* Include peppers, onions, mushrooms, tomatoes and spinach in your breakfast eggs (scrambled, omelet, etc.). Add kale, spinach, carrots, cucumbers and lettuce to "green" shakes or protein shakes. Snack on cold baby carrots, cherry tomatoes, celery, cucumbers and broccoli either alone or with low-calorie dressings/dips. Prepare stir fry meals with an assortment of your favorite vegetables (we enjoy broccoli, peppers and onions).

- *Consume a small-medium sized salad prior to eating lunch and/or dinner.*

Be sure to minimize extra calories by using low-calorie dressings and adding croutons sparingly. This can a tremendous help to prevent overeating especially in combination with increased water consumption around meal times.

- *Get creative with what foods you are cooking.* If you are someone who gets bored of eating the same meals over and over, look to other resources for new and healthy recipe ideas (i.e. health blogger's websites or Pinterest pages, health-oriented magazines, etc.). If practicing this, be sure you keep the habits in mind, and remember that not all recipes that are marketed as "healthy" are truly healthy for you. Many people are in the same boat as you and enjoy providing recipes that have helped them succeed.

HABIT #5: EAT MORE PROTEIN

Increase your daily protein intake so that you are consuming one of the following three amounts/totals each day (pick what works best for you):

- *A protein source (poultry, red meat, fish, eggs) roughly the size of your fist with each meal.*

- *Roughly 30-40 grams of protein from a protein rich food (meat, fish, eggs, soy products, Greek yogurt or cottage cheese) with each meal.*

- *An approximate daily protein total of 0.75 gram of protein per 1 lb. of body weight (ex: if you weigh 160 lbs., you will aim to consume roughly 120 total grams of protein per day – multiply your weight by 0.75).*

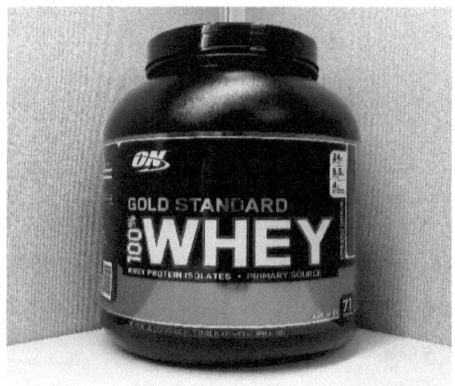

Consuming a sufficient amount of protein will be key to maximizing your weight loss efforts. Protein is a very important macronutrient that has a ton of benefits, especially for those looking to lose weight. Protein keeps you feeling fuller longer and helps you feel more satiated after a meal. This helps reduce hunger and cravings, ultimately decreasing how many calories you're consuming. It also helps you build muscle and retain muscle mass when calories are being lowered. It is important for recovery from your workouts, and it helps increase strength and improves bone density. Finally, protein has a greater "thermic effect of food" than carbohydrates or fats as your body will burn more calories digesting it than the other macronutrients (high protein diets have been shown to boost metabolism by 80 to 100 calories per day). Protein is hands down the most important macronutrient for weight loss, so you need make sure you're eating a sufficient amount of it each day!

Barring any food allergies, you should aim to consume a variety of whole foods to meet your protein requirements each day. This means eating a good mix of fish, poultry, lean beef, nuts, beans, eggs, certain dairy products, etc. Do your best to get the majority of your protein from whole food sources, but feel free to use any protein supplements as needed to reach your daily totals (one whey/soy/hemp protein shake each day is totally fine). Also utilize resources such as the MyFitnessPal phone app, NutritionData.self.com and CalorieKing.com along with reading nutrition labels to get a better understanding of just how much protein is in the foods you eat. Not only do we want you to develop this habit, but we also want you to gain a better understanding of exactly what you consume each day.

Presented below is a chart that highlights the protein content of many popular "high protein" foods. This should help give you a better understanding of what foods you can choose to increase your daily protein intake.

Food	Amount	Protein (grams)	Food	Amount	Protein (grams)
Meats (Cooked)			**Dairy**		
Low Fat Meats (poultry, beef, pork)		8	Greek Yogurt	2/3 Cup	15
Fattier Meats	1 ounce	7	Cottage Cheese	1/2 Cup	14
Fish		8	Milk	1 Cup	8
Shrimp		6	Cheese	1 Ounce	5-8
Meats (Uncooked)			**Legumes**		
Chicken Breast		24	Black Beans	1 Cup	15
Ground Beef		23	Soy Beans	1 Cup	28
Lean Ground Turkey	4 ounces	21	Green Peas	1 Cup	8
Fish		20	Lentils	1 Cup	18
Shrimp		16	Peanuts	1 Ounce	8
Eggs			**Other**		
Large Egg	1	6	Quinoa	1 Cup	8
Egg White (form large egg)	1	4	Pumpkin Seeds	1 Cup	12
Liquid Egg Whites	1/2 Cup	12	Ezekiel Bread	1 Slice	4

With this habit, we list three separate options that will all result in higher protein consumption. Choose the option that you think you can stick to the best and feel free to experiment with it. Like all of the other habits, progress slowly and do not try to completely overhaul your diet in one shot. Slow steady progress is what will result in long term sustainable results.

Tips to increase adherence:
- *Snack smarter.* Most people choose to snack on foods that contain plenty of carbs and very little protein. Instead of choosing chips, crackers, snack bars, and pretzels try cheddar or cottage cheese, Greek yogurt, almonds, lean jerky, nuts

or peanut butter with fruit.

- *Add extra protein to your meals.* Get creative and see where you can drop a few additional protein packed ingredients into the foods you love. Chopped almonds sprinkled in salads, yogurt and oatmeal works well. Add some turkey, chicken, salmon, tuna and/or cheese to your salads. Beans are an excellent addition to many foods if you're looking for a plant based protein food to add. Just make sure you don't overdo things and end up adding a large amount of additional calories in the process. Keep the portions reasonable and eat until you feel full/satisfied.

HABIT #6: EAT MODERATE FAT

Keep your daily fat intake moderate by utilizing one of the following methods:

- **Consume approximately 15-25 grams of fat with each meal**

- **Consume approximately 30% of your daily calories from fat (appropriately portioned into your meals throughout the day)**

Eating the correct amount of fat with each meal will be very helpful for those looking to lose weight and improve their hunger management. When your meals contain a moderate amount of fat, you are better able to achieve and maintain fullness as well as keep your appetite controlled for longer periods of time (compared to protein and carbohydrate). Dietary fat helps slow down how quickly your stomach empties food after a meal and it causes your body to release hormones that signal satiety (hunger satisfaction) and appetite suppression. When you consume a sufficient level of fat you will likely be able to make it much longer between meals and avoid being hit with overwhelming hunger. The key is to make sure that your fat intake is not too low or too high, but moderate! If it is too low, hunger will reappear much sooner than you would like. If it is too high, you will consume excess calories and sabotage your weight loss efforts.

The range of 15 to 25 grams per meal is recommended as it should allow you to get roughly 30% of your total daily calories from fat (moderate fat intake) if 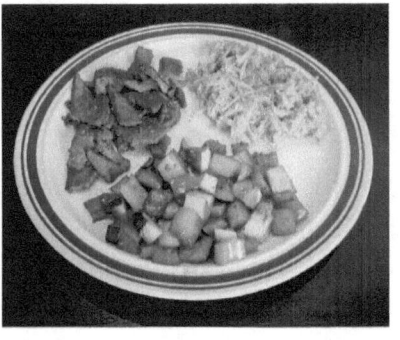 you eat the recommended three to four meals per day. The ideal daily fat intake for most people is around 30% of total calories (in line with the American Heart Association's guidelines) to support health and leanness. Low fat diets typically offer less appetite satisfaction and can cause drops in blood sugar leading to excessive hunger and the potential to over-snack. In the long term, low fat diets have been shown to be ineffective for those looking to keep off the initial weight they lost from dieting. High fat diets have been shown to fail in the long term as well due to the potential to overshoot your daily calories (fat is very calorically dense; one gram of fat contains nine calories compared to protein and carbohydrate which contain four calories per gram). Consistent high fat intake can also weaken your body's sensitivity to the hormones that are necessary to feel satisfied after a meal.

The bottom line: Research has shown that your best chance to lose weight and keep it off long term is to keep your daily fat consumption moderate. Low fat and high fat diets have been shown to be more difficult to maintain and decrease your chances of successful long term weight management.

Please understand that you will not have to measure every single gram of fat that you eat or strictly stick to the recommendations above. This habit should serve as a general guideline for discovering just how much fat you need in your diet to help you lose weight and better manage your hunger. Practice reading nutrition labels and understanding just how much fat is in the foods you enjoy. Experiment with different types/amounts of fat to see what helps you stay the fullest between meals (without consuming excess calories). As with the other habits, this takes practice and is a learning process so be patient. Over time, this will become second nature to you.

In terms fat types, aim to consume primarily Monounsaturated fats (avocado, nuts, olives, olive oil), Polyunsaturated Omega-3 fats (seafood, flaxseed, walnuts, canola oil, soybean oil) and Saturated fats (meats, milk, cheese, coconut oil, cocoa butter). Try to avoid consuming Trans fats whenever possible.

THE HABIT SYSTEM

Presented below is a table displaying many popular "high fat" foods that you can start including in your meals to meet your daily fat requirements.

Food	Amount	Fat (grams)
Dairy		
Plain Yogurt	1 Cup	8
American Cheese	1 Slice	3
Cheddar Cheese	1 Slice	9
Cottage Cheese	1 Cup	9
Nuts		
Almonds		15
Cashews		13
Macadamia	1 Ounce	21
Pecans		21
Pistachios		13
Walnuts		18
Oils		
Olive Oil		14
Coconut Oil	1 Tbsp	14
Peanut Oil		14

Food	Amount	Fat (grams)
Vegetables		
Avocado	1	29
Green Olives	1 Ounce	4
Black Olives		4
Animal Products		
Large Egg	1	5
Ground Beef		6
Rib Eye Steak		8
New York Strip Steak	1 Ounce	4
Salmon		3
Mackerel		4
Seeds		
Chia Seeds		9
Flax Seeds	1 Ounce	12
Pumpkin Seeds		13
Sunflower Seeds		14

HABIT #7: REDUCE LIQUID CALORIES

Reduce your overall consumption of beverages that contain calories (milk, juice, soda, sweetened tea, sports drinks, energy drinks, alcoholic beverages, etc.).

Identifying where all of your daily calories are coming from is incredibly important for your fat loss efforts. Drinking sugar/fat filled liquids throughout the day can add a substantial amount of calories to your diet that do very little to help keep you feeling full. You are much better off getting your calories from nutrient dense, whole foods that will keep you full, satisfied and energized for hours. You are going to fight off hunger for much longer with a 400 calorie meal instead of a 400 calorie Starbucks drink. It is time to start getting your calories from better sources!

First work on identifying just how many liquid calories you consume throughout the day (utilize the Food Journal habit for this). Then, slowly work on reducing these liquid calories or eliminating them altogether if you feel you can handle that level of reduction. Think of liquid calories as the "low hanging fruit" of your fat loss efforts. With the large variety of different low sugar/low calorie drink options that are available in today's market place, there really are no good reasons to consume the full sugar versions. We understand taste plays a big role in people's beverage choices, but start experimenting with low calorie alternatives and find what tastes the best for you.

Do your best to gradually reduce the total amount of liquid calories you consume each day. If there is a particular drink that you absolutely cannot do without, practice measuring and controlling portions of that beverage. Be mindful of exactly how many calories they contain and do your best to drink them sparingly.

Tips to increase adherence:
- *Be sure to pay attention to how many smoothies/shakes you consume and what is in them, even if they are full of*

"healthy" items. People often do not realize how quickly calorie totals add up, especially when you start adding in multiple ingredients. We suggest either keeping your smoothies/shakes as simple as possible with only the essential foods/ liquids/powders you need or limiting the total amount of smoothies/shakes you consume each week. Keep in mind, whole food meals will keep you fuller longer so do your best to opt for those first.

- *Similar to the prior tip, be mindful of exactly what you put in your daily coffee.* Between sugar, milk, syrups and creamers, it is easy to rack up a pretty significant amount of calories in just one 8 to 16 ounce beverage. Practice utilizing low calorie/calorie free sweeteners and creamers instead. If you absolutely cannot find any low calorie alternatives that you enjoy, work on measuring and reducing portion sizes. Instead of three cups of coffee per day with unmeasured amounts of sugar and creamer, see if you can operate on two cups with one teaspoon of sugar and two tablespoons of half and half (as an example).

- *Keep track of how many alcoholic beverages you consume each week.* People often do not realize just how many calories their wine, beer or mixed drinks contain but those calories can add up pretty quickly as well. Please understand that you do not need to cut alcoholic beverages out of your diet completely. Asking you to do so would be unreasonable and unless your goal is to compete in a physique/bodybuilding competition, it's likely unnecessary. One major component of long term dieting success is relying on balance instead of total restriction. Begin tracking just how many alcoholic drinks you consume each week so that you at least know what your starting point is. Depending on the level of success you're experiencing with the other habits, decide on whether you realistically need to alter your alcohol consumption. If you're losing weight with the other nine habits and really enjoy drinking four alcoholic beverages on

Habit #7: Reduce Liquid Calories
Reach Your "Satisfaction Zone"

Saturday nights, continue doing so. If you feel that you'd like to accelerate your results however, and you can manage to drink three beverages instead of four, do so.

HABIT #8: DRINK MORE WATER

Increase your daily water consumption so that you are consuming no less than 64 ounces per day (roughly 2 liters).

Water is an excellent tool to utilize when you are working to lose fat. Studies have shown that drinking water can boost metabolism by 24 - 30% over a period of 60-90 minutes, helping you burn a few additional calories. Drinking more water throughout the day will help keep you hydrated (especially important when following an exercise program) and can replace calorie packed drinks. Drinking more will also help keep you feeling fuller longer and can help reduce the feeling of hunger when a meal is not readily available. We highly recommend drinking a full glass of water before and/or with each of your meals if possible. This will help you feel full more quickly and may help prevent you from overeating. One study concluded that drinking 17 ounces of water roughly 30 minutes before meals helped dieters eat fewer calories and lose 44% more weight.

Tips to increase adherence:

- Keep a bottle of water with you at all times throughout the day. Studies have shown (and common sense would lead you to believe) that proximity helps increase water intake. You are going to drink more water if there is a bottle of it on your desk as opposed to having to walk to a water fountain.

- Practice set daily habits such as drinking a full glass of water first thing in the morning and making sure you finish a full glass with each meal. Commit to drinking a full bottle with each workout. Reminders on your phone may provide further help if you need them.

HABIT #9: IMPROVE YOUR SLEEP & RECOVERY

Prioritize getting sufficient sleep and adequate recovery from your workouts using the tips below.

One major factor that is often neglected in many people's fat loss journey is sufficient sleep and recovery. While the primary driver of weight loss is a calorie deficit (burning more calories than you are consuming), other important factors come into play that can undermine your efforts if they are not addressed. If you are not getting enough sleep each night you may be setting your fat loss progress back tremendously.

Lack of sleep has been associated with obesity and weight gain. A large study in 2005 that included over 9,500 adults suggested that the rising obesity epidemic in the United States may be caused in part by a decrease in the average number of sleep hours. The study demonstrated that individuals between the ages of 32 and 49 years who slept less than seven hours each night had higher average body mass indexes and were more likely to be obese than those that slept over seven hours. The study also demonstrated that staying awake beyond midnight seemed to also increase the likelihood of obesity.

Not getting sufficient sleep each night can negatively affect the hormones in your body that regulate appetite. Lack of sleep increases levels of the hormone that stimulates hunger (Ghrelin) and decreases levels of the hormone that suppresses appetite (Leptin). Sleep deprivation also raises levels of Cortisol, the stress hormone frequently associated with fat gain. The combination of these three changes sets you up to consume excess calories and store them as fat by being significantly hungrier and less satisfied after your meals.

Lack of sleep can also negatively affect your ability to recover from workouts and decrease your energy to complete subsequent workouts.

THE HABIT SYSTEM

Sleep deprivation decreases protein synthesis (how your body grows muscle) and can lead to higher incidences of injury. Working out is hard enough for most people, but being exhausted makes it much more difficult especially if you continue to remain in sleep debt.

As a general rule of thumb, most people need about 7-9 hours of sleep each night for adequate recovery. The following tips can be used to help improve your recovery and ensure that you are getting an appropriate amount of sleep each night. Similar to the previous habits, start with one or two reasonable action items and slowly build from there. Trying to completely overhaul your habits in one shot is difficult for most people so work at whatever pace feels best for you.

1. Reduce or eliminate stimulants (caffeine/ nicotine) altogether beginning in the afternoon each day. Stimulants can negatively affect sleep if they are consumed less than six hours prior to bedtime.

2. Avoid consuming alcohol before bed. Alcohol disrupts the normal rhythms of sleep and decreases the amount of time

people spend in REM sleep. Some people use alcohol to help them get to sleep quicker however the amount of sleep disruption experienced in the second half of your night can offset the benefits in the first half.

3. Keep the temperature in your bedroom cool. The available research indicates that a temperature between 60 and 67 degrees Fahrenheit is optimal for sleep. Temperatures above 75 degrees and below 54 degrees can be disruptive to sleep.

4. Avoid large, heavy meals close to bed time. Being overly full and trying to digest a large meal can disrupt your sleep. Opt for a light meal if you need to eat close to bed time.

5. Keep your bedroom as dark as possible. Avoiding light (even the dull glow of your electronics) can help better manage your circadian rhythms. Bright light triggers our brains to be awake and alert, so avoid it the best you can around bed time.

6. Avoid noise by keeping your bedroom as quiet as possible (remove noisy electronics and ticking watches/clocks) or add some type of white noise (fans, humidifiers and white noise apps work very well).

7. Use a consistent daily routine to help wind down before bed time. Your body needs time to get into sleep mode so engage in some type of calming activity such as reading, yoga, meditation, aroma therapy or breathing exercises. Also try to keep a relatively consistent sleep and wake time even on weekends if possible.

8. Write whatever thoughts, worries or concerns you have down on paper to help clear your mind of the clutter that can hinder your sleep. Writing out your to-do list for the next day can also help relieve any anxiety that may keep you up at night.

HABIT #10: FOLLOW THE "LEAN MEAL" FORMULA TO CREATE YOUR MEALS

Use the following structure to create the majority of your meals each week.

- *A lean protein source (poultry, fish, red meat, eggs, soy) roughly the size of your fist*

- *Several handfuls of vegetables*

- *One to two handfuls of starchy carbohydrates and/or fruit*

- *Moderate amount of fat (from foods and/or toppings/dressings/oil)*

- *Low calorie beverage or water*

The final habit provides you with a useful structure to help you put the previous habits into action. The "Lean Meal" formula can be used as a checklist to ensure that your meals are geared towards fat loss as this type of meal composition allows you to consume a ton of quality nutrients, control/reduce your caloric intake and feel more full/satiated after you eat. This structure will help ingrain better eating habits and can serve as a standard eating guide to be used in the future.

Please understand that you can also use variations of this formula to create lean meals that might not exactly resemble the meal pictured below. Lunch for example, may be comprised of a homemade tuna salad sandwich on 100% whole wheat or whole grain bread topped with baby spinach, tomato and onion with an apple on the side. This meal contains sufficient protein from the tuna and bread, moderate fat from the mayonnaise and tuna, a small serving of vegetables from the toppings and a reasonable amount of quality carbohydrates from the bread and apple. Breakfast may be comprised of a three egg omelet containing one and a half cup of chopped vegetables and two slices of American cheese with one cup of fruit on the side. This meal contains plenty of protein and fat from the eggs and cheese, a decent serving of vegetables and a reasonable amount of quality carbohydrates from fruit.

Get creative and design meals that you will enjoy and look forward to. Eating bland meals that lack flavor and will not satisfy you is not necessary for weight loss. Instead rely on thoughtful planning and ask yourself the following questions when creating each meal for the week:

- Does this meal contain enough protein to keep me satisfied after I've eaten it?

- Does this meal contain moderate fat that will help me stay full for hours?

- Did I include enough vegetables to add more volume to my meal?

- Did I include foods that I actually enjoy eating?

THE HABIT SYSTEM

While it would be ideal to follow this structure seven days per week, you will likely experience much success even if you are only able to follow it for five days each week. Based on the average person's weekly schedule, following this structure Sunday through mid-Friday and eating a few "off plan" meals/snacks during the remaining time should work just fine. Do your best to keep those off plan meals reasonable though. Many people make the mistake of using their "cheat meals" as an excuse to enjoy as many high calorie foods as they possibly can. Instead of completely overindulging and consuming a ton of excess calories, apply Habit 3 by eating slowly and stopping once you reach your satisfaction zone. You can still enjoy the foods you love but by applying this system of habits you can minimize the negative affects it may have on your weight loss efforts.

When creating your meals, be sure to select your protein source first and your vegetables second. These two components are what your meals should be built around. Once you have done that, fill in the remaining space on your plate with a reasonable amount of carbohydrates and fats. This ensures that your main focus is on the foods that are going to make the most fat loss impact (protein and veggies) and not on the foods that people typically over-eat and subsequently consume excess calories from.

Tips to increase adherence:

- As with the previous habits, slow and steady implementation is going to be key. Practice following this structure with one meal at a time. Once you are able to consistently follow the structure with that meal, add an additional meal. Continue adding days until you reach 5 - 7 days per week.

- Utilize the tips presented in Habit 2 in conjunction with this structure to properly prepare your meals for the week. Preparation is especially important to making this habit successful.

CONCLUDING THOUGHTS

World renowned strength coach Dan John made an excellent point about diet and exercise programs when he stated that "Everything works for about six weeks.". Why? Because he is absolutely correct. Nearly all popular diets and workout programs will deliver visible results within the first six weeks for those that can properly follow them. When you introduce a new routine that is much different from what you typically do, your body tends to respond fairly quickly. New stimulus often produces new results. Unfortunately though, if you cannot turn this new stimulus into a sustainable lifestyle your results are likely going to be very short lived. As we highlighted at the beginning of this book, dieting failure rates are incredibly high as are post-diet weight regains primarily due to the short term focus many people have. We need to take a different approach to dieting.

The Habit System was created to help you learn what habits are most important for losing fat and maintaining an ideal body weight. The system is a set of general dieting rules that you can follow for the rest of your life. Crash dieting is going to cause more frustration than benefit and there are no magic supplements that can lose the fat for you. Your secret dieting weapon is practice and consistency, two key components the Habit System was built around.

Be patient, focus on consistency and understand that your fitness journey is lifelong. Put your best effort into tackling the system head on but still make time to enjoy the foods and activities you love! Dieting shouldn't be a miserable process that deprives you of the things you truly enjoy in life, so do not allow it to be.

You **will** reach your fitness goals.

You **will** improve your body composition and health. You **will** make progress.

Let's get started.

ACKNOWLEDGEMENTS

First and most importantly, thank you to my other half Lauren and my parents Keith and Denise for their constant love and encouragement. Without their support, this book would not exist. Thank you to all of the clients who have put their trust in me over the years to help them reach their goals, especially Elyse Royer and Dennis Hood. Finally, a tremendous thank you to all of my friends and family who have believed in me and given me the strength to pursue my passion.

THE HABIT SYSTEM

REFERENCES

Andrade AM, et al. "Eating slowly led to decreases in energy intake within meals in healthy women." *J Clin Endocrinol Metab.* 2010 Jan;95(1):333-7.

Begg DP, et al. "The endocrinology of food intake." *Nat Rev Endocrinol.* 2013 Oct;9(10):584-97.

Beglinger C. "Fat in the intestine as a regulator of appetite-role of CCK." *Physiol Behav.* 2004 Dec 20;83(4):617-21.

Boeing H, et al. "Critical review: vegetables and fruit in the prevention of chronic diseases." *Eur J Nutr.* 2012 Sep; 51(6): 637-663.

Boshmann M, et al. "Water Drinking Induces Thermogenesis through Osmosensitive Mechanisms." *Obesity (Silver Spring).* 2010 Feb;18(2):300-7.

Camilleri M. "Peripheral mechanisms in appetite regulation." *Gastroenterology*. 2015 May; 148(6): 1219-1233.

Cavallo DN, et al. "Adult intake of minimally processed fruits and vegetables: Associations with cardiometabolic disease risk factors." *J Acad Nutr Diet*. 2016 May 10. Pii: S2212-2672(16)30108-3.

Dennis EA, et al. "Water consumption increases weight loss during a hypocaloric diet intervention in middle-aged and older adults." *Obesity (Silver Spring)*. 2010 Feb;18(2):300-7.

Dougkas A, et al. "Protein-enriched liquid preloads varying in macronutrient content modulate appetite and appetite-regulating hormones in healthy adults." *J Nutr*. 2016 Mar;146(3):637-45.

Drake C; Roehrs T; Shambroom J; Roth T. "Caffeine effects on sleep taken 0, 3, or 6 hours before going to bed." *J Clin Sleep Med* 2013;9(11):1195-1200.

Duffey KJ, et al. "Modeling the effect of replacing sugar-sweetened beverage consumption with water on energy intake, HBI score and obesity prevalence." *Nutrients.* 2016 Jun 28;8(7). Pii: E395.

Eklund D, et al. "Fitness, body composition and blood lipids following 3 concurrent strength and endurance training modes." *Appl Physiol Nutr Metab.* 2016 Jul;41(7):767-74.

Gangwisch JE; Malaspina D; Boden-Albala B et al. "Inadequate sleep as a risk factor for obesity: analyses of the NHANES I." *SLEEP* 2005; 28(10):1289-1296.

GORGO Fitness Magazine. "How To Lose Fat and Keep It Off – By Dr Layne Norton." Online video clip. YouTube. YouTube, 10 Oct 2014. Web.

Grodstein F, et al. "Three-year follow-up of participants in a commercial weight loss program. Can you keep it off?" *Arch Intern Med.* 1996 Jun 24;156(12):1302-6.

Howard CE, Porzelius LK "The role of dieting in binge eating disorder: Etiology and treatment implications" *Clin Psychol Rev.* 1999 Jan;19(1):25-44.

Hu FB. "Are refined carbohydrates worse than saturated fat?" *Am J Clin Nutr.* 2010 Jun;91(6):1541-2.

Kim MK, et al. "Fast eating speed increases the risk of endoscopic erosive gastritis in Korean adults." *Korean J Fam Med.* 2015 Nov; 36(6): 300-304.

Kokkinos A, et al. "Eating slowly increases the postprandial response of the anorexigenic gut hormones, peptide YY and glucagon-like peptide-1." *J Clin Endocrinol Metab.* 2003 Dec;88(12):6015-9.

Korkeila M, et al. "Weight-loss attempts and risks of major weight gain: a prospective study in Finnish adults." *Am J Clin Nutr.* 1999 Dec;70(6):965-75.

Kreider RB, et al. "Protein for exercise and recovery." *Phys Sportsmed.* 2009 Jun;37(2):13-21.

Lappaleinen R, et al. "Drinking water with a meal: a simple method of coping with feelings of hunger, satiety and desire to eat." *Eur J Clin Nutr.* 1993 Nov;47(11):815-9.

Little T, et al. "Oral and gastrointestinal sensing of dietary fat and appetite regulation in humans: modification by diet and obesity." *Front Neurosci.* 2010; 4:178.

Lowe MR, et al. "Dieting and restrained eating as prospective predictors of weight gain." *Front. Psychol.* 4:577.

Lowe MR. "Dieting: proxy or cause of future weight gain?" *Obes Rev.* 2015 Feb;16 Suppl 1:19-24.

Markwald R, et al. "Impact of insufficient sleep on total daily energy expenditure, food intake, and weight gain." *Proc Natl Acad Sci USA.* 2013 Apr 2; 110(14): 5695-5700.

McManus K, et al. "A randomized controlled trial of a moderate-fat, low-energy diet compared with a low fat, low-energy diet for weight loss in overweight adults." *Int J Obes Relat Metab Disord.* 2001 Oct;25(10: 1503-11.

Moghettie P, et al. "Metabolic effects of exercise." *Front Horm Res.* 2016;47:44-57.

Monteiro CA, et al. "Increasing consumption of ultra-processed foods and likely impact on human health: evidence from Brazil." *Public Health Nutr.* 2011 Jan;14(1):5-13.

Ohlsson B, et al. "Modification of a traditional breakfast leads to increased satiety along with attenuated plasma increments of glucose, C-peptide, insulin, and glucose-dependent insulinotropic polypeptide in humans." *Journal of Nutrition Research* 36.4 (2016): 359-368.

Onen SH, Onen F, Bailly D, Parquet P. "Prevention and treatment of sleep disorders through regulation of sleeping habits." *Presse Med.*1994; Mar 12; 23(10): 485-9.

O'Reilly GA, et al. "Mindfulness-based interventions for obesity-related eating behaviors: A literature review." *Obes Rev.* 2014 Jun; 15(6): 453-461.

Orwell S, Frank K. "Fat-Burner – Scientific Review on Usage, Dosage, Side Effects." *Examine.com.* 15 Nov 2012. Web.

Pesta DH, et al. "A high-protein diet for reducing body fat: mechanisms and possible caveats." *Nutr Metab (Lond)*. 2014 Nov 19;11(1):53.

Piovezan RD, et al. "The impact of sleep on age-related sarcopenia: Possible connections and clinical implications." *Ageing Res Rev* 2015 Sep;23(Pt B):210-20.

Reddy NL, et al. "Enhanced thermic effect of food, postprandial NEFA suppression and raised adiponectin in obese women who eat slowly." *Clin Endocrinol (Oxf)*. 2015 Jun;82(6):837-7.

Ruffault A, et al. "Randomized controlled trial of a 12-month computerized mindfulness-based intervention for obese patients with binge eating disorder: The MindOb study protocol." *Contemp Clin Trials*. 2016 Jun 29;49:126-133.

Shai I, et al. "Weight loss with a low-carbohydrate, Mediterranean, or low-fat diet." *N Engl J Med*. 2008; 359:229-241.

Smith CF, et al. "Flexible vs. rigid dieting strategies: relationship with adverse behavioral outcomes." *Appetite*. 1999 Jun;32(3):295-305.

Spiegel K, et al. "Brief communication: Sleep curtailment in healthy young men is associated with decreased leptin levels, elevated ghrelin levels, and increased hunger and appetite." *Ann Intern Med* 141 (2004): 846-850.

Sutton EF, et al. "No evidence for metabolic adaptation in thermic effect of food by dietary protein." *Obesity (Silver Spring)*. 2016 Jun 29. Doi: 10.1002/oby.21541. [Epub ahead of print]

Tan Y, et al. "Relationships between Sleep Behaviors and Unintentional Injury in Southern Chinese School-Aged Children: A Population-Based Study." *Int J Environ Res Public Health*. 2015 Oct 16;12(10):12999-3015.

Tanumihardjo SA, et al. "Strategies to increase vegetable or reduce energy and fat intake induce weight loss in adults." *Exp Biol Med (Maywood)*. 2009 May;234(5):542-52.

Veldhorst MA, et al. "Presence or absence of carbohydrates and the proportion of fat in a high-protein diet affect appetite suppression but not energy expenditure in normal-weight human subjects fed in energy balance."Am J

Clin Nutr. 2009 Sep;90(3):519-26.

Veldhorst MA, et al. "Gluconeogenesis and energy expenditure after a high-protein, carbohydrate-free diet."
J Am Diet Assoc. 2008 Jul;108(7):1186-91.

Voronoa RD, et al. "Overweight and obese patients in a primary care population report less sleep than patients with a normal body mass index." *Arch Intern Med* 2005;165:25-30.

Weigle DS, et al. "A high-protein diet induces sustained reductions in appetite, ad libitum caloric intake, and body weight despite compensatory changes in diurnal plasma leptin and ghrelin concentrations." *Br J Nutr.* 2010 Nov;104(9):1395-405.

WORKSHEETS

THE HABIT SYSTEM

HABIT LOG

Date:												
Habit #1: Food Journal												
Notes:												
Habit #2: Prepare!												
Notes:												
Habit #3: Eat Slowly, Stop at Satisfaction Zone												
Notes:												
Habit #4: Eat More Vegetables												
Notes:												
Habit #5: Eat More Protein												
Notes:												
Habit #6: Eat Moderate Fat												
Notes:												
Habit #7: Reduce Liquid Calories												
Notes:												
Habit #8: Drink More Water												
Notes:												
Habit #9: Improve Your Sleep & Recovery												
Notes:												
Habit #10: Follow the "Lean Meal" Formula												
Notes:												

FOOD JOURNAL

Meal (Include time)	Food/Beverage (Type and amount)	Calories	Protein (Grams)	Carbs (Grams)	Fat (Grams)	Notes
				Meals		
	Meal Notes:					
	Meal Notes:					
	Meal Notes:					
	Meal Notes:					
					Snacks	
	Meal Notes:					
	Meal Notes:					
	Meal Notes: